WEIGHT LOSS AFTER MENOPAUSE:

The Essential Guide to Healthy Weight Loss After Menopause

Ryan Karl

Table Of Content

Chapter 1: Introduction

Joan had always been a bit overweight, but it wasn't until she was in her late 40s that she started to feel the effects of it. She was constantly tired, had difficulty sleeping, and found herself craving unhealthy snacks more than ever. Despite her best efforts, she couldn't seem to lose weight.

One day, while browsing the shelves in her local bookstore, Joan came across a book entitled Weight Loss After Menopause: The Essential Guide to Healthy Weight Loss After Menopause. She skimmed through the pages and quickly realized how beneficial this book could be for her.

Joan decided to give the book a try and soon, she was armed with the knowledge and techniques to begin her journey to a healthier weight. She learned about the various diet plans and exercise routines that were most effective for her age group. She also read about the importance of getting enough rest and reducing stress levels.

To her delight, Joan started to see results within a few weeks. By the end of the first month, she had lost 10 pounds. She was so proud of her progress and felt more energetic than she had in years.

As she continued to follow the advice and tips from the book, Joan continued to lose weight and improve her overall health. She was able to keep the weight off and maintain a healthy lifestyle.

Weight Loss After Menopause was truly a blessing for Joan. It not only helped her to lose weight, but it also gave her the confidence to live a healthier life. She was finally able to look in the mirror and feel proud of what she saw. She was truly a success story.

As women enter their 40s and 50s, they often experience changes in their bodies due to the natural process of menopause. It's common for women to gain weight during this time, and it can be difficult to find the right combination of nutrition, exercise, lifestyle, and emotional support to help them lose weight and keep it off.

This guide is designed to provide women with the information they need to understand the causes of weight gain during menopause, as well as the best strategies for healthy and sustainable weight loss. By following the steps outlined in this guide, women will be able to find the combination of diet, exercise, and lifestyle changes that will help them achieve their weight loss goals while also maintaining their overall health and well-being.

Chapter 2: Understanding Menopause and Weight Gain

All women go through menopause naturally at some time in their life. Physical and emotional changes are occurring during this time, and there may also be a few unforeseen difficulties. Weight gain is one of the most typical problems that women have throughout menopause.

There are several causes of weight increase during menopause. Menopause-related hormonal changes can result in a loss of muscle mass and an increase in fat. The result might be an increase in total body weight. Additionally, estrogen levels decrease after menopause. This may increase hunger and food desires, which might ultimately result in weight gain.

Women can take a few steps to prevent or minimize weight gain during menopause. Priority one should be given to maintaining a healthy diet and exercise routine. A balanced diet full of fruits, vegetables, healthy grains, and lean meats can help prevent weight gain. Another crucial component of maintaining health throughout menopause is exercise. Regular exercise can aid in maintaining muscle mass and burning calories, which can aid in controlling weight.

Additionally, it's critical to obtain enough rest throughout menopause. A rise in hunger hormones brought on by sleep deprivation may result in overeating and weight gain. To maintain a healthy balance in your hormones, aim for seven to eight hours of sleep each night.

Finally, it's critical to control your stress levels throughout menopause. Cortisol levels rising as a result of stress might boost hunger and desire for unhealthful meals. Maintaining healthy cortisol levels can be accomplished by learning stress management techniques like yoga and meditation.

Women can make the required lifestyle modifications to maintain their weight by being aware of the link between menopause and weight gain. Women can lessen the effects of menopause on their weight by maintaining a healthy diet, engaging in regular exercise, and managing their stress.

Chapter 3: Causes of Weight Gain During Menopause

Now that you understand the role hormones and physical changes play in menopause-related weight gain, it's important to consider the other factors that can contribute to weight gain during this life stage.

While some weight gain during menopause is normal, there are a few primary causes that can lead to excessive weight gain. Knowing what these are can help you take steps to manage your weight and maintain your overall health during this time.

1. **Hormonal Changes:** During menopause, the body's production of the hormones estrogen and progesterone begins to decline, leading to a decrease in metabolism and an increase in fat storage. This can result in weight gain, particularly in the abdomen, hips, and thighs.

2. **Insulin Resistance:** As menopause progresses, the body's sensitivity to insulin, a hormone that helps regulate blood sugar levels, decreases. This means that blood sugar levels remain high, leading to increased food cravings and weight gain.

3. **Stress:** Stress can cause the body to produce more of the hormone cortisol, which can lead to increased fat storage, especially in the abdominal area.

4. **Poor Diet:** Eating a diet high in processed foods and low in nutrient-rich fruits, vegetables, and whole grains can cause weight gain.

5. **Lack of Exercise:** Exercise helps boost metabolism and burn calories, so a lack of physical activity can lead to weight gain.

6. **Sleep Deprivation:** Not getting enough sleep can lead to hormone imbalances that can cause weight gain.

7. **Medications:** Some medications, such as antidepressants and corticosteroids, can lead to weight gain.

8. **Age:** As we age, our metabolism naturally slows down, leading to weight gain.

9. **Genetics:** Genetics can play a role in weight gain, as some people are more prone to storing fat than others.

10. **Alcohol:** Drinking alcohol can lead to weight gain, as it is high in calories and can disrupt the body's hormones.

By understanding the causes of weight gain during menopause, you can take steps to manage your weight and maintain your overall health. Eating a healthy, balanced diet, exercising regularly, getting enough sleep, and limiting alcohol consumption are all important steps to take. Additionally, speaking to your doctor about any medications you may be taking can help ensure that they are not contributing to weight gain.

Chapter 4: Nutrition and Diet Strategies for Healthy Weight Loss After Menopause

To achieve and maintain healthy weight loss after menopause, it's important to focus on nutrition and diet. Eating a balanced diet full of whole foods can help you feel fuller for longer and can also help you maintain your energy levels throughout the day.

When it comes to nutrition, the key is to focus on nutrient-dense foods that are high in fiber and protein. These types of foods will help you feel fuller for longer and will provide your body with the energy it needs to function properly.

Luckily, there are a variety of nutrition and diet strategies that can help women to maintain a healthy weight after menopause. Here are 10 nutrition and diet strategies for healthy weight loss after menopause.

1. **Eat plenty of fruits and vegetables:** Fruits and vegetables are packed with vitamins and minerals, and they are low in calories. Eating plenty of fruits and vegetables can help to keep you full and can help you to reach your daily nutritional goals.

2. **Limit processed and packaged foods:** Processed and packaged foods tend to be high in calories, fat, and sugar. They can also lack the same nutritional value as fresh produce. Limiting these foods can help you to maintain a healthy weight.

3. **Avoid added sugars:** Added sugars are found in many processed and packaged foods. They can contribute to weight gain and can also increase your risk for chronic diseases. Avoiding added sugars can help you to maintain a healthy weight.

4. **Eat protein-rich foods:** Protein-rich foods can help to keep you full and can also help to maintain muscle mass as you age. Eating lean

proteins such as fish, poultry, and beans can help you to reach your daily nutritional goals.

5. **Increase fiber intake:** Fiber can help to keep you full and can also help to lower your cholesterol levels. Eating plenty of fiber-rich foods such as whole grains, fruits, and vegetables can help to keep your weight in check.

6. **Drink plenty of water:** Water can help to keep you full and can also help to flush out toxins from your body. Drinking plenty of water can help to keep your body hydrated and can help to promote weight loss.

7. **Limit your alcohol intake:** Alcohol can be high in calories and can also contribute to weight gain. Limiting your alcohol intake can help to keep your weight in check.

8. **Get enough sleep:** Getting enough sleep can help to reduce stress and can also help to keep

your weight in check. Aim to get 7-8 hours of sleep each night.

9. **Monitor your portion sizes:** Eating smaller portions can help to reduce your calorie intake and can also help to keep your weight in check. Use smaller plates and bowls to help you to monitor your portion sizes.

These 9 nutrition and diet strategies can help you to maintain a healthy weight after menopause. Eating a balanced diet and getting enough exercise can help you to stay fit and healthy as you age.

Chapter 5: Exercise Strategies for Weight Loss After Menopause

Exercise is an important part of maintaining a healthy lifestyle, especially for women entering or in menopause. It can help to manage symptoms such as hot flashes, night sweats, and mood swings, as well as reduce the risk of developing certain diseases like osteoporosis and heart disease. It can also be an effective strategy for weight loss after menopause. Here are some exercise strategies that can help you reach your weight loss goals.

1. **Focus on Strength Training:** Strength training is an important part of any exercise program, and it can be especially beneficial for weight loss after menopause. It helps to build lean muscle mass, which boosts your metabolism and helps you burn more calories

throughout the day. Aim to do two to three strength training sessions per week, focusing on major muscle groups like your legs, chest, back, and arms.

2. **Add Interval Training:** Interval training is a great way to get your heart rate up and burn more calories in less time. It involves alternating between short bursts of high intensity and longer periods of lower intensity. Try to do a few interval training sessions per week, such as running sprints or cycling intervals.

3. **Include Cardio:** Cardio exercises like running, walking, swimming, and biking are great for weight loss after menopause. Aim to do at least 30 minutes of moderate-intensity cardio three to five times per week.

4. **Try Yoga and Pilates:** Yoga and Pilates can be great tools for weight loss after menopause. They help to strengthen and tone your muscles, while also improving your flexibility and

balance. Aim to do at least one session of yoga or Pilates per week.

5. **Get Moving Throughout the Day:** It's important to stay active throughout the day, not just during your workouts. Incorporate more movement into your day by taking the stairs instead of the elevator, parking further away from the entrance, and taking a walk during your lunch break.

These are just a few exercise strategies that can help with weight loss after menopause. It's important to find an exercise regimen that works for you and that you enjoy doing. With a combination of strength training, interval training, cardio, yoga, Pilates, and regular daily activity, you can reach your weight loss goals and stay healthy.

Chapter 6: Stress Management and Mental Well-Being After Menopause

One of the most important things a woman can do to manage stress and maintain mental health during and after menopause is to nurture herself. Self-care is essential during this time and can include things such as getting enough rest, exercising regularly, and managing stress levels. It's also important to stay connected with friends and family, as social support can be invaluable during this period.

In addition to focusing on nutrition and exercise, it's also important to pay attention to your mental health and well-being when it comes to weight loss. Stress can have a negative impact on your weight loss efforts, as it can lead to the release of hormones that can increase appetite and lead to overeating.

It's important to take steps to reduce stress in your life, such as getting enough sleep, engaging in relaxation activities, and spending time with friends and family. Additionally, yoga, meditation, and other forms of mindfulness can all help you reduce stress and maintain your mental well-being.

It's also important to remember that weight loss is a journey, and it's important to be patient and kind to yourself throughout the process. Achieving a healthy weight can take time, and it's important to celebrate the small successes along the way.

Chapter 7: Supplements and Alternative Therapies for Weight Loss After Menopause

Supplements for Weight Loss After Menopause

There are several types of supplements available to help women lose weight. These include herbal supplements, fiber supplements, vitamins, minerals, probiotics, and essential oils. Each of these has its unique benefits when it comes to weight loss.

Herbal Supplements

Herbal supplements are a popular choice for those looking to lose weight after menopause. Many herbs have been used for centuries to aid in weight loss. Some of the most popular herbs for weight loss include green tea, ginger, cayenne pepper, and turmeric.

Green tea extract is a powerful antioxidant that has been found to help with weight loss. It helps to increase the body's metabolism and burn more calories, which can lead to weight loss.

These herbs help to boost the metabolism and reduce appetite. They can also help to reduce inflammation, which can lead to weight loss.

Fiber Supplements

Fiber is an important part of a healthy diet and may help with weight loss after menopause. Fiber helps to keep you feeling full for longer periods and increases the rate at which food is digested. It can also help reduce cholesterol levels, which can help with weight loss.

Vitamins and Minerals

Vitamins and minerals are essential for maintaining a healthy weight. Certain vitamins and minerals, such as Vitamin D, calcium, and zinc, can help to boost metabolism and reduce appetite.

Omega-3 fatty acids are polyunsaturated fats that are found in fish, nuts, and certain vegetable oils. They have been found to reduce inflammation and have beneficial effects on the cardiovascular system. They may also help reduce body fat, particularly in the abdominal area.

They can also help to regulate blood sugar levels, which can reduce cravings and help to keep cravings in check.

Probiotics

Probiotics are beneficial bacteria that help to maintain a healthy digestive system and are naturally found in the gut. They improve digestion by maintaining a healthy balance of bacteria found in the gut thereby helping with weight loss

They can also help to reduce inflammation and support weight loss. Probiotics are found in certain foods, such as yogurt, kefir, and fermented vegetables.

Essential Oils

Essential oils are another popular option for those looking to lose weight. Certain essential oils, such as peppermint and grapefruit, can help to reduce cravings and boost metabolism. They can also help to reduce stress levels, which can lead to weight gain.

It's important to talk to your doctor before taking any supplements, as some can have adverse effects or interact with certain medications.

Alternative Therapies for Weight Loss After Menopause

In addition to dietary supplements, several alternative therapies may help with weight loss after menopause. Some of the most known therapies include:

1. **Acupuncture:** Acupuncture is an ancient Chinese practice that involves the insertion of thin needles into certain points of the body. It is believed to help balance the body's energy and may help reduce stress, which can lead to weight loss.

2. **Herbal Remedies:** Herbal remedies are made from plants and have been used for centuries to treat a variety of illnesses. Some herbal remedies may help with weight loss after menopause by increasing the body's metabolism and reducing appetite.

3. **Hypnosis:** Hypnosis is a state of deep relaxation in which a person is more open to suggestions. It has been used to help people change bad habits, such as overeating, and may help with weight loss after menopause.

Benefits of Supplements and Alternative Therapies

There are many benefits of using supplements and alternative therapies to aid in weight loss. These include:

Increased metabolism: Certain supplements, such as green tea and ginger, can help to boost metabolism. This can lead to increased calorie burning, which can lead to weight loss.

Reduced cravings: Some supplements, such as probiotics and essential oils, can help to reduce cravings. This can lead to fewer calories consumed, which can help to promote weight loss.

Improved digestion: Certain supplements, such as probiotics, can help to improve digestion.

This can lead to increased nutrient absorption, which can help to support weight loss.

Reduced inflammation: Some supplements, such as turmeric, can help to reduce inflammation. Inflammation can lead to weight gain, so reducing inflammation can help to support weight loss.

In addition to focusing on nutrition, exercise, and mental well-being, there are also certain supplements and alternative therapies that can help you achieve your weight loss goals. Certain supplements, such as omega-3 fatty acids, can help reduce inflammation in the body, while certain herbs and botanicals can help boost your metabolism and reduce cravings.

Chapter 8: Putting It All Together: A Healthy Weight Loss Plan for Menopause

Now that you understand the different aspects of weight loss after menopause, it's time to put it all together and create a healthy weight loss plan. The key to successful weight loss is to find the right combination of nutrition, exercise, lifestyle, and emotional support that works for you.

Weight loss during menopause can be a challenge. Hormonal changes, lifestyle issues, and age-related health issues can all make it difficult to shed those extra pounds. But, with a little planning, you can create a healthy weight loss plan for menopause that will help you reach your goals.

The first step in creating a healthy weight loss plan for menopause is to determine your current body weight and body composition. This can be done through a variety of methods, such as body mass index (BMI), waist circumference, and body fat percentage. Knowing your current body weight and composition can help you set realistic goals and plan for gradual, sustainable weight loss.

Next, it's important to create an eating plan that is tailored to your individual needs. Menopausal women may benefit from eating smaller meals throughout the day, as well as avoiding processed and sugary foods. Pay attention to portion sizes and limit your intake of processed foods and added sugars. A diet rich in fiber, lean proteins, and healthy fats can help you feel fuller and longer and provide the nutrients necessary for optimal health.

In addition to eating right, regular physical activity is key for successful weight loss. Exercise not only helps to burn calories, but it can also help to reduce stress, boost energy levels, and improve your overall health. When it comes to exercise, focus on activities that you enjoy and that won't put too much strain on your body. Aim to get at least 30 minutes of exercise per day, and make sure to take breaks when you need them.

Choose activities that you enjoy, such as walking, biking, swimming, or yoga, and aim to get at least 30 minutes of exercise each day.

Finally, it's important to stay motivated and on track with your weight loss goals. Make sure to track your progress and celebrate your successes, no matter how small.

Pay attention to your mental health and well-being. Take steps to reduce stress in your life, and remember to be patient and kind to yourself throughout the process.

You can also join a weight loss support group or online community to share tips and encouragement with other menopausal women.

Weight loss after menopause can be challenging, but it is possible. By following the steps outlined in this guide, you can create a healthy weight loss plan that works for you. Remember to focus on nutrition, exercise, lifestyle, and mental well-being, and you will be well on your way to achieving your weight loss goals.

Chapter 9: Conclusion

My goal in writing this book was to provide readers with the essential information they need to know to safely and successfully achieve healthy weight loss after menopause. We have discussed the physiological and psychological changes that occur during menopause and the importance of finding the right kind of nutrition for your body. We have also discussed the importance of engaging in regular physical activity and the potential health benefits that come from doing so. Finally, we have discussed the importance of having realistic expectations and taking the time to develop a plan that works for you.

I hope that this book has been helpful and that it has provided readers with the information they need to make informed decisions about their health and well-being and has inspired readers to take charge of their health and make positive lifestyle changes to achieve their health and weight loss goals. Menopause is a time of transition and change and it can be overwhelming and confusing at times. However, with the right knowledge, motivation, and support, it is possible to successfully manage the changes that menopause brings and to achieve healthy and sustainable weight loss.

I wish all of my readers the best of luck in achieving their health and weight loss goals. Thank you for taking the time to read this book and for considering my advice. I hope that you have enjoyed the journey and that you have a healthier and happier future ahead of you.

www.ingramcontent.com/pod-product-compliance
Lightning Source LLC
Chambersburg PA
CBHW051722250726
48653CB00008B/3144